# EASY HEALTHCARE:

# OBAMACARE

By

# Lori-Ann Rickard

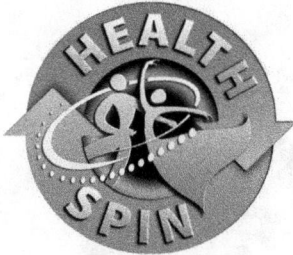

Presented by
Expert Health Press

ISBN-10: 1940767075

ISBN-13: 978-1-940767-07-9

*To Bridget,*
*for your expertise and support.*

# TABLE OF CONTENTS

# INTRODUCTION

The **Affordable Care Act**, otherwise known as **ObamaCare**, transformed healthcare in the United States, and it continues to have a significant impact on individuals' lives every day. The question of whether that impact is positive or negative is a hotly debated topic, but answering that question is not the point of this guide. Instead, we'll give you a practical breakdown of what the law contains and what it means to you: what has changed, how it has changed, and if those changes are relevant to you or your loved ones.

## *Why Is It Called "ObamaCare?"*

Many people are confused by the different names used to describe the same thing. The official name is the **Patient Protection and Affordable Care Act (ACA),** which was signed into law by President Obama on March 23, 2010. Because passing the law was a central goal of the president's administration, the law quickly got the nickname "ObamaCare." Others may refer to it as ACA, the Affordable Care Act, or "health reform." All of these terms are referencing the same law.

ObamaCare is a giant, complex law that has ten separate large sections with many subparts and hundreds of provisions. The law made major changes to health insurance, which will be implemented over time. These changes have been hotly debated in the media; however, the law also contains several sections that have not received much attention, such as those addressing childhood obesity, drug development, and nursing home care, among others.

So what are the 10 things you need to know about ObamaCare?

# 1.

# What Did ObamaCare Change First?

When the law was passed in 2010, it made many immediate changes to how health insurance works. Prior to 2010, health insurance companies generally could make what many considered to be unfair rules that benefited them financially, but hurt individual policy holders. You might have periodically heard stories about health insurance companies unfairly denying coverage when a patient needed it most, or employees who could not change jobs due to the likelihood of losing their insurance. ObamaCare attempted to outlaw some of these unfair practices.

## No More Denials for Children's Pre-Existing Conditions

One of the first changes prevented insurance companies from denying children coverage due to **pre-existing conditions.** A pre-existing condition is a health problem you have before you apply for insurance. For example, if your child was born with a serious birth defect, the child may need care throughout his or her life. Prior to ObamaCare, if the parent changed health insurance plans, the new insurance provider could refuse to cover the child due to the pre-existing condition. ObamaCare immediately prohibited this practice by insurance companies.

## No More Denials for Technical Errors

Another change the law made in 2010 was to prohibit insurance companies denying coverage for a patient due to a technical error in their health insurance application. Prior to ObamaCare, insurance companies could, for example, review a breast cancer patient's insurance application, and, if they found a minor error, use that error to deny coverage. This common practice was immediately banned in 2010.

## NO MORE DENIALS FOR HITTING A "LIFETIME LIMIT"

Another common practice among healthcare insurers involved placing a **lifetime limit** on every insured person. In other words, the insurance company would pay up to a certain maximum dollar amount on an individual, and once that limit was reached, end coverage. So, if you had a long-term illness such as cancer, it was very likely you would quickly hit your lifetime limit and be denied healthcare coverage even though you were still paying your monthly premiums. Being treated for cancer is expensive and insurance companies wanted to limit the uncontrolled costs these patients presented. However, insurance companies under ObamaCare are now no longer allowed to have lifetime limits on policies.

## IF YOU ARE DENIED COVERAGE, YOU CAN APPEAL TO AN EXTERNAL SOURCE

In 2010, ObamaCare created a new way for patients to appeal a denial of coverage by an insurance company. Prior to ObamaCare, insurance companies could deny coverage and the only recourse for the patient was to ask the insurance company to review its own decision. It's not surprising that the insurance company would rarely, if ever, reverse its denial. These denials could often occur when a patient needed coverage the most, such as for bone marrow transplants or other expensive, life-saving treatments.

Under ObamaCare, denials must now be evaluated by external review panels. Health plans must retain certified healthcare review organizations in order to provide external oversight and case evaluation. Certified healthcare specialists run these external review panels. The patient can seek an external review to make sure the insurance company is not denying them coverage due to unfair reasons.

## PREVENTATIVE CARE COVERED

Prior to ObamaCare, many health insurance plans focused only on covering you when you got sick and did not offer to pay for **preventative care.** Preventative care includes annual physicals and health screenings such as colonoscopies and mammograms. Because the costs were not covered, many individuals did not take these steps, which can keep you healthier longer and identify serious illnesses before they become life threatening. Upon the passing of ObamaCare, health plans were required to cover preventive care without additional cost to the patient, such as co-pays or deductibles.

## YOUNG ADULTS COVERED UNDER A PARENT'S INSURANCE

Another big change allowed children up to the age of 26 to stay covered under a parent's insurance plan. They do not have to live at home or be in school to be covered. Prior to ObamaCare, health insurance companies did not have to provide coverage for children under their parent's policy after they reached the age of 18, even if they were in school or lived at home. Due to the economic downturn of 2008 and beyond, many young adults had difficulty securing jobs and could not easily obtain their own health insurance. With ObamaCare, young adults can retain their health insurance coverage through their parents while they pursue additional training or education or accept a job without health insurance to acquire valuable experience to move ahead in the work force.

# THE BOTTOM LINE...

- Insurance companies can no longer deny coverage to children who have pre-existing conditions.

- Insurance companies can do longer deny insurance coverage due to technical errors on applications.

- Insurance companies can no longer put life-time limits on insurance coverage.

- If you are denied coverage, you can now appeal the denial to an external review board.

- You will now have coverage for preventative care services.

- Children are able to remain on their parent's insurance until the age of 26.

# 2.

# WHAT SHOULD SENIORS KNOW ABOUT OBAMACARE?

As the law rolled out, ObamaCare made other significant changes that would affect seniors. Some of the changes focus on adding more coverage for seniors.

### PRESCRIPTION DRUG DISCOUNTS AND WELL VISITS FOR SENIORS

**Medicare** is the federal government insurance program that provides health coverage to people over the age of 65. Medicare also provides coverage for people with certain disabilities as well as those with end stage renal disease. Medicare Part A covers hospital and skilled nursing stays as well as hospice and some home healthcare. Medicare Part B covers doctors' services, outpatient services, and medical supplies. Medicare Part C governs the Medicare Advantage Plans, which is type of Medicare run by private insurance companies. Medicare Part D covers prescription drugs.

Prior to ObamaCare, Medicare Part D covered prescription drug costs for seniors up to a certain set amount each year. Many seniors take a multitude of drugs and so often reached a point where drugs would no longer be paid for the rest of the year. In 2014, this coverage gap occurs after the senior (through his or her deductible) and Medicare pay a set amount of $2,850. This number can change depending on the year. This coverage gap is also referred to as the "**donut hole**." Once the senior hits the coverage gap, drug companies charge seniors an exorbitant cost, which they often cannot afford. In 2014, ObamaCare mandated that the coverage gap ends when costs for a senior exceeds $4,550. While the senior is in the coverage gap, ObamaCare implemented a 50 percent discount for prescription brand-name drugs covered by Medicare Part D and a 20 percent discount on generic brands. ObamaCare abolishes the "donut hole" altogether in 2020. ObamaCare also provided for annual wellness checkups for seniors.

## HIGH RISK SENIORS GET SPECIAL ATTENTION

After a hospital admission, seniors often leave the hospital only to return within 30 days for the same problem. This sometimes occurs because he or she does not have adequate follow-up care, or may have limited transportation to get to follow-up appointments with their doctor or pick up prescriptions from the pharmacy. The **Community Care Transitions Plan (CCTP)** implemented under ObamaCare went into effect in 2011 and will run for five years. It helps to keep high-risk Medicare patients from returning to the hospital by connecting them with services in their communities such as a home health agency.

## HIGH INCOME SENIORS PAY MORE

Under ObamaCare, high-income individuals receiving Medicare will be required to pay more for their Medicare Part B premium, which covers physician and outpatient services. A Medicare beneficiary earning more than $85,000 ($170,000 for a couple) will be required to pay a higher premium. High-income Medicare beneficiaries will also be required to pay more for prescription drug coverage under Medicare Part D. These income thresholds will remain the same through 2019.

## EQUALITY BETWEEN MEDICARE AND MEDICARE ADVANTAGE PLANS

ObamaCare also focuses on eliminating costs from **Medicare Advantage** plans. Medicare Advantage is health insurance offered to seniors by private companies, which is approved by Medicare. Before the passage of ObamaCare, the federal government paid $1,000 more per person to those private companies for coverage under a Medicare Advantage plan than traditional Medicare. This increased cost was then passed on to all Medicare beneficiaries. ObamaCare decreases some of the payments to the companies offering Medicare Advantage plans in order to level the playing field for all Medicare beneficiaries. This change does not affect Medicare beneficiaries, only the private companies that provide Medicare Advantage health plans.

## No "Death Panels" or Rationing

Seniors can often hear the terms "death panels" or "rationing" in the media debate surrounding ObamaCare. Opponents to ObamaCare will refer to a panel of experts who have the power to deny care to critically ill seniors, or the expectation that certain procedures for seniors, such as knee or hip replacement surgery, will no longer be approved after you reach a certain age. Both concepts are false.

ObamaCare has a provision that allows the appointment of an **Independent Payment Advisory Board (IPAB)**, which is a 15-member group made up of non-practicing physicians, healthcare policy experts, healthcare facilities managers, health service researchers, employers, consumers, and representatives for the elderly. This board has limited authority to make proposals designed to curb the overall cost of Medicare if it becomes uncontrollable. However, the IPAB is specifically barred from recommending cuts to healthcare that threaten Medicare beneficiaries' access to care. ObamaCare specifically states that the IPAB may not engage in rationing.

Additionally, because healthcare costs have been decreasing, the IPAB has not even formed as of 2014. Even if it is formed, the board has very limited authority, and it does not have the ability to deny healthcare under any circumstances.

# THE BOTTOM LINE...

- Seniors now have coverage for well visits.

- Seniors now receive prescription drug discounts when they hit the coverage gap under Medicare Part D.

- Special plans have been established for seniors who are at risk for hospital readmissions.

- Payments made to Medicare Advantage Plans were lowered to more closely align with Medicare.

- High income seniors will pay more for Medicare.

- ObamaCare does NOT set up "death panels."

- Obamacare does NOT ration care for seniors.

# 3.

# WHAT DOES OBAMACARE MEAN FOR INSURANCE PLANS AND HEALTHCARE PROVIDERS?

## HEALTH INSURANCE COMPANIES MUST SPEND 85 PERCENT OF THEIR FUNDS ON HEALTHCARE

Another provision in ObamaCare ensures that health insurance plans use most of their funds to pay for healthcare services. This seems fairly obvious but many insurance companies had previously focused large amounts of their premium dollars on "administrative costs" (in other words, business expenses that also included lucrative salaries for executives). ObamaCare requires that 85 percent of all premium dollars be spent by health insurance companies on healthcare services or health quality initiatives in large group markets, which includes companies with 50 employees or more. In small group markets covering employers with 49 employees or less, the insurance company must spend 80 percent of its premium dollars on healthcare. If the health insurance company's administrative costs or profits are too high, the insurance company must give money back to consumers.

## NO DISCRIMINATION BASED ON HEALTH STATUS OR GENDER

Beginning in 2014, insurance companies are prohibited from charging higher insurance rates due to a patient's health status or gender. Prior to this ObamaCare requirement, insurance companies regularly charged different people different rates depending on how much the insurance company predicted the person's health coverage would cost. The insurance companies used statistics to determine how much a woman might cost to insure versus a man. Insurance rates regularly varied drastically based on these statistics.

Also, prior to ObamaCare, some insurance companies denied coverage to people who choose to participate in a **clinical trial.** A clinical trial is a research study that uses human participants to answer specific health questions. Those questions might include whether or not a new treatment works for a certain disease or how weight gain affects your heart. Clinical trials play a key role in getting new drugs and medical devices approved for use, and can be the fastest and safest way to find treatments that work for those patients who have not responded to currently available options. Clinical trials are often used to discover new cancer treatments and treatments for other life-threatening illnesses. Patients were often discouraged from participating in clinical trials because insurance companies later denied their health insurance coverage. This practice is no longer allowed under ObamaCare.

## Moving Away from "Fee for Service" Payments

In 2015, payments to physicians will change from "**fee for service**" to payments based on the value of the care provided. If physicians can show that they have improved the outcomes for their patients, they will receive more reimbursement for the care they provide. Traditionally, physicians charge a "fee" for each service they provide. A patient is charged a fee for an office visit, a procedure, a test, etc. In the future, physicians will have to show that they improved the condition of the patient to get payment rather than simply charging a patient for each task they perform regardless of outcome.

## Hospitals Get Incentive Payments

Hospitals are normally paid a certain sum based on the specific illness the patient is diagnosed with upon admission to the hospital. For example, if you are admitted to a hospital for pneumonia, insurance companies pay the hospital a set amount for that illness. In 2012, ObamaCare incentivized hospitals with additional payments from the federal government if they improved quality and lowered costs during that hospital stay. The government listed specific illnesses and asked hospitals to report their progress. For the first time, hospitals openly reported heart attacks, heart failure, pneumonia, surgical care and infections. Since 2012, hospitals report to the federal government how well they take care of patients who have had heart attacks. How many patients lived and died? How long did patients with these conditions stay in the hospital? How many patients got infections and what kind? All of this information is now available to the public. In the coming years, hospitals will be incentivized to release other information that will help patients receive better care at a lower cost.

This payment structure shifts the focus from only paying health-care providers to treat sick patients to improving the outcomes for those patients. This is a big change in healthcare. Previously, health-care providers benefited financially only when patients were sick. Switching to a payment system that is partially based on improving patient outcomes encourages healthcare providers to get patients well and keep them well.

## ACCOUNTABLE CARE ORGANIZATIONS CREATED

**Accountable Care Organizations ("ACOs")** were also intro-duced in 2012 as a part of the Medicare program. An ACO is a group of physicians who join together to improve treatment qual-ity and better coordinate care. If the ACO is able to reduce costs as a result of that coordination, its members can share in the savings it generates. Again, this incentivizes doctors differently since histori-cally they have been paid only when a patient is sick and had no financial reason to coordinate care. Coordination is absolutely nec-essary since patients often have many health problems and many physicians. With Accountable Care Organizations, physicians now have that motivation.

## MORE ELECTRONIC HEALTH RECORDS

ObamaCare encourages healthcare providers to move away from traditional paper medical records toward **electronic health records (EHRs)**. ObamaCare implemented many new regulations for health plans that require the transfer of patient information in a secure and confidential manner. Electronic exchange of health data makes the exchange of healthcare information simpler and faster. This switch to electronic records alleviates some administrative burdens and costs while at the same time increases quality and decreases medical errors.

In 2012, another law, the **Recovery and Reinvestment Act**, provided that if physicians adopted the first stage of an electronic health record, they would receive an incentive of $44,000. This incentive caused millions of physicians to convert to electronic health records. In 2014, more than 70 percent of physicians said they are using EHRs.

### PAYMENT FOR AN "EPISODE" OF CARE

Another implemented change involves Medicare paying a **"flat rate payment"** to a hospital, group of healthcare providers, and post-acute care facilities for an "episode" of care for a patient. Medicare will now pay the healthcare providers one fee for a patient's care. Once again, this is a change from paying healthcare providers in a fragmented manner based on the services they provide to a payment system that encourages all providers to work together to get the patient better and improve his or her quality of care. This change pays providers as a "team" so that they are financially encouraged to design care around the best patient outcomes. Many private insurance companies are following this model and moving away from "fee for service" payments.

### PRIMARY CARE DOCTORS GET A PAYMENT INCREASE

Primary care doctors also saw an increase in their payments for **Medicaid** patient care. The law requires that all primary care doctors receive 100 percent of Medicare rates for caring for Medicaid patients. Normally, Medicaid pays significantly less than Medicare. This increased payment is fully funded by the federal government and encourages doctors to see Medicaid patients.

# THE BOTTOM LINE...

- Health insurance companies must now spend 85 percent of their premium dollars on patients and improving quality of care.

- Insurance companies can no longer discriminate based on gender or health status.

- Healthcare providers will increasingly be paid based on patient outcomes and not just on providing a service.

- Hospitals can receive incentive payments if they improve quality of care and lower costs.

- Accountable Care Organizations created by ObamaCare incentivize doctors to coordinate patient care.

- Electronic heath records are now required to promote efficiency and decrease medical errors.

- Medicare will begin paying healthcare providers as a team for a patient's "episode of care" rather paying multiple "fees for service."

- Medicaid payments to primary care doctors will be raised to the same level as Medicare payments.

# 4.

# WHO MUST BUY
# INSURANCE NOW?

## Very Few People Will Have to Buy Insurance

ObamaCare mandates that all U.S. citizens, with very few exceptions, must have insurance or face a penalty. For those who do not currently have insurance, the law created healthcare exchanges to allow the uninsured to shop for and purchase insurance. But, surprisingly, most people will never sign up for coverage on those exchanges.

Forty-eight percent of the U.S. population has employer-sponsored health insurance. Medicare covers another 15 percent. Medicaid accounts for an additional 15 percent. Other government health insurance programs cover 2 percent of the population, and another 5 percent of the population participates in non-group plans. Thus, only 15 percent of the U.S. population is currently uninsured. Therefore, most people will never need the exchanges created as a result of ObamaCare.

Those who will need those plans are the remaining 20 percent of Americans who are uninsured (15 percent) or who normally buy their insurance in the individual health plan market (5 percent). It's important to note, however, that caring for the uninsured affects everyone, even the insured. Because healthcare personnel must provide emergency healthcare without regard to the person's ability to pay for the services, everyone pays for the cost of the uninsured. Hospitals and healthcare providers must raise their fees to cover the cost of uncompensated care and remain in business. If, for example, Starbucks had to provide free coffee to those who could not pay, their prices for paying customers would soon become insanely high and they would quickly go out of business.

## Will Seniors Lose Their Medicare Coverage?

The simple answer is "no." Further, if you are a senior, it is important to know that you are covered by Medicare, and you do not need to buy insurance on the exchanges. A number of scams have arisen involving the elderly that attempt to confuse seniors about their health insurance and collect "fees" to help them "enroll in ObamaCare." This can be especially confusing because the enrollment period for choosing a Medicare plan may be similar to the enrollment period for plans created for the ObamaCare exchanges. If you over 65, you do not need to "enroll in ObamaCare." Nor will you have to pay any penalty for not having insurance since you are covered by Medicare.

Seniors should also be aware that health insurance exchanges do not sell "Medigap" policies, which supplement the coverage seniors get through Medicare. Therefore, seniors should not look for health insurance coverage on the health exchanges.

The only situation when a senior would be eligible to shop for insurance on the exchanges is if he or she is retired and is covered by their former employer's health insurance and not Medicare. They are entitled to purchase on the health exchange if the health exchange coverage is cheaper than the employer's coverage. However, the senior will not be entitled to any tax subsidy for the health exchange insurance coverage.

## How Much Will ObamaCare Coverage Cost?

The cost of coverage for an ObamaCare health plan will vary widely depending on three major factors: your age, your income, and where you live. ObamaCare allows health insurance companies to charge significantly more for an older shopper compared to a young shopper. For example, a health plan for a 58-year-old can cost three times more then the same health plan for a 23-year-old. The reason for this is that the health insurance company expects to pay far more for the 58-year-old's healthcare then for a young, healthy 23-year-old. It is also true that in certain parts of the country healthcare costs are more than in other parts of the country. Additionally, for people who earn less than four times the poverty level (about $47,000 for an individual or $96,000 for a family of four), they will be entitled to subsidies, which may pay for the entire cost of the monthly premium.

Each ObamaCare health plan will have some costs which the person will have to pay for themselves. These are called "**out-of-pocket**" costs. "Out-of-pocket" costs will vary depending on which health plan you choose. If you qualify for Medicaid, your "out-of-pocket" costs will be almost nothing. Also, for some low-income families, there are protections that limit "out-of-pocket" costs.

## KNOW YOUR TERMS

There are numerous terms you should understand prior to shopping for insurance. First, you will be asked to pay a monthly **premium**. The premium is the monthly price you pay to have access to the insurance plan. The next term you need to understand is co-pay. A **co-pay** is a specific flat fee you pay when you go to see a doctor. The co-pay remains the same no matter how much the doctor charges.

Next, you need to know what is **"in network"** and what is **"out of network."** Each insurance plan has doctors and hospitals that are in the health plan's network. If you see one of these doctors, you are "in network" and the charge will be less than a doctor who is not in the health plan's network. If you go to your own doctor who is not in the network of the health plan, you are "out of network" and you will pay more of the cost of seeing the doctor. For example, if your "in network" co-pay for a doctor's visit is $15, you will pay that amount each time you visit a doctor who is "in network." If you see a doctor who is "out of the network," your co-pay can be significantly higher.

The next term to be aware of is **deductible**. A deductible is the amount you have to spend before your insurance company starts making payments for your healthcare. Some services–for example preventative care–are exempt from the deductible and are offered at no cost immediately to you no matter how high your deductible is.

**Coinsurance** is similar to a co-pay; however, it is a percentage of the cost of the actual procedure as opposed to a flat fee.

The last term that is commonly used is **out-of-pocket maximum.** An out-of-pocket maximum is the absolute most you will have to spend on your healthcare in a year. For most plans, the out-of-pocket maximum is set by federal law at $6,350 for an individual; $12,700 for a family. The rule regarding out-of-pocket maximum amounts listed above were delayed from being implemented from 2014 to 2015. Therefore, until 2015, there is no limit on how much you might pay for these non-covered items.

## THE BOTTOM LINE...

- Only 15-20 percent of the U.S. population will have to buy healthcare as a result of ObamaCare.

- Seniors are not required to purchase insurance under ObamaCare. They are covered by Medicare.

- The average cost of insurance on the healthcare exchanges will vary depending on your age, location, and income.

- When shopping for insurance plans on the exchanges review the terms used to define policies.

# 5.

# WHAT IS A HEALTH EXCHANGE?

## FEDERAL HEALTHCARE EXCHANGE MARKETPLACE

**Health insurance exchanges** became available in 2013. A "healthcare exchange" or "marketplace" is an online site where you can shop for insurance. On October 1, 2013, the federal healthcare exchange, www.healthcare.gov, opened, and, although major technical issues plagued the site for months to come, it marked the first time people could go online and search a wide range of health insurance options in one place. On this exchange and the state-sponsored ones that followed, individuals can easily compare plans and rates, something that was nearly impossible to do previously, since most companies kept their rates private or actively discouraged comparisons. Now, like going to Amazon or any other online shopping site, users can dynamically compare prices and pick the plan that is right for them.

### STATE HEALTH EXCHANGES V. FEDERAL HEALTH EXCHANGE

Under ObamaCare, states could either set up their own exchange or have residents use the federal health insurance exchange. Some states choose to have their own exchange, share an exchange with another state, or have a joint-run healthcare exchange with the federal government. These states are Arkansas, California, Colorado, Connecticut, Delaware, District of Columbia, Hawaii, Idaho, Illinois, Iowa, Kentucky, Maryland, Massachusetts, Michigan, Minnesota, Nevada, New Hampshire, New Mexico, New York, Oregon, Rhode Island, Utah, Vermont, Washington, and West Virginia.

The remaining states have decided not to develop health exchanges. Thus, the majority of states are using the federally run healthcare exchange. If your state does not have an exchange, you can use the federal healthcare exchange to shop for coverage. However, if your state runs its own health exchange, you will need to enroll through your state-run health exchange. If you are trying to locate your state-run exchange, you can always start at www.health-care.gov and it will direct you to your state-run exchange.

Some state-run exchanges have been running particularly smoothly, such as Connecticut, Kentucky, Washington, and Rhode Island. However, others have faced issues, among them Hawaii, Oregon, Maryland, and Vermont.

## WHAT DO YOU NEED TO GET STARTED?

First, understand what your status is. Are you younger than 65 and not eligible for Medicaid? Are you unemployed and without insurance? Are you self-employed and without insurance? Does your employer not offer health insurance? In all of these circumstances, you can shop for insurance on a health insurance exchange.

In order to purchase health insurance from a health exchange, you will need some basic information about you and your family. You will need ages and social security numbers. If you have doctors or hospitals you want to continue to use, make sure you have their names nearby for reference so you can check on the exchange to see if they participate in any of the plans you consider. Before making a final decision, always call your doctor's office to make sure they accept the health plan you are considering.

# THE BOTTOM LINE...

- The federal government operates a nationwide healthcare exchange at www.healthcare.gov.

- Many states operate their own exchanges.

- If your state runs its own health exchange, you must use that health exchange.

- If your work does not provide health insurance, you are able to shop for insurance on health exchange.

- You will need some basic information about you and your family in order to enroll on health exchange, including ages and social security numbers.

- Before enrolling, call your healthcare providers to determine which health plans they participate in.

# 6.

# HOW DO I CHOOSE A HEALTH PLAN ON THE HEALTH EXCHANGE?

You should consider a number of factors when you're shopping for health insurance on the exchanges.

## ALL INSURANCE PLANS COVER "BASIC SERVICES"

In the past when you shopped for insurance, finding out what specific services a plan covered was nearly impossible. Often, you would purchase a policy and find out later that many of necessary services or treatments were not covered or required exorbitant deductibles or co-pays.

Under ObamaCare, every plan must cover certain basic services, so they can be taken for granted when you sign on. First, all plans will cover ambulatory services, which include doctor visits, clinic visits, and same-day surgery. All plans will also provide coverage for home care and hospice, although some plans will limit the coverage to 45 days.

Second, every plan will cover emergency services, including the cost of an ambulance. You cannot be penalized for going out of network or not receiving prior authorization for an emergency. Third, you will receive coverage for hospitalization. All the services provided in a hospitalization will be covered. You will also receive coverage for a stay in a skilled nursing facility, though the covered stay may be limited to 45 days.

Additionally, you will receive coverage for laboratory services when a doctor orders a test to diagnose a problem or illness. You are also covered for preventative laboratory tests such as screenings for breast or prostate cancer.

All plans must also cover maternity care and newborn care. This includes coverage for care during your pregnancy. This benefit was often excluded from prior health plans or had to be purchased separately.

Another basic benefit is coverage for mental health services and addiction treatment. This coverage is for both inpatient and outpatient care and includes substance abuse. Substance abuse, however, may only be covered for up to 20 days per year. Rehabilitation and rehabilitation devices are also a basic benefit. Plans must cover 30 visits per year for both physical and occupational therapy. Speech therapy is also covered for 30 visits per year. Cardiac and pulmonary rehabilitation is also covered for 30 visits per year.

Pediatric services are also a basic covered service under ObamaCare. Well check ups along with recommended vaccines and immunizations are covered for infants and children. Dental and vision care must also be offered for children younger than 19. This coverage includes two routine dental exams, an eye exam, and corrective lenses each year.

Prescription drugs are also covered as a basic service under ObamaCare. Preventative and wellness services for adults are also a basic covered service under ObamaCare. Physicals, immunizations, and screenings designed to prevent and detect certain medical conditions are covered.

Lastly, care for chronic conditions, such as asthma and diabetes are basic covered services. Certain preventative services are covered at 100 percent. You will not owe a co-pay or coinsurance even if you have not yet met your yearly deductible. These services are covered at 100 percent as long as you receive this service within your network. Preventative services include:

- Alcohol misuse screening and counseling

- Aspirin used to prevent cardiovascular disease

- Cholesterol screening

- Colorectal cancer screening

- Adult depression screening

- Type II diabetes screening

- Diet counseling for adults at risk

- HIV screening for individuals between the ages of 15-65

- Adult immunization vaccines including hepatitis A, hepatitis B, shingles, HPV, flu, measles, mumps, rubella, meningococcal, pneumonia, tetanus, diphtheria, pertussis (Td/Tdap), and chickenpox vaccines.

## EXCEPTIONS FOR INSURANCE PLANS NOT PURCHASED THROUGH AN EXCHANGE

It is important to note that some insurance plans that are not purchased from a health exchange will not include these basic services. Fully insured large group plans, self-funded plans and grandfathered plans (those that were in existence on March 23, 2010) are not required to include essential health benefits. Large group plans include insurance plans such as General Motors or Citibank health insurance plans. Self-funded plans are those plans which are paid for directly by the employer instead of the employer purchasing their health insurance from an outside insurance company such as UnitedHealthcare. The federal government also allowed an extension for all health plans that do not contain these basic services to continue through 2016 as long as their own state allows those plans to continue. Some states have agreed to the extension of the non-compliant plans and other states have not.

## WHAT PLAN DO I CHOOSE?

When an individual is looking to select the health insurance coverage that is right for themselves and their family, the healthcare exchange provides five categories to help make the choice more clear. The categories are: Bronze, Silver, Gold, Platinum, and Catastrophic.

A **Bronze plan** will be the cheapest plan and will split covered expenses 60-40. This means that for all covered services the health insurance company will pay 60 percent of the costs and you will have to pay the remaining 40 percent. The Bronze plan will also have the most basic benefits and will likely have the most limited network of doctors and hospitals. The Bronze plan was designed for those who will likely not need much healthcare.

The **Silver plan** splits all covered expenses 70-30. Again, this means that for all covered services the health insurance company will pay 70 percent of the costs and you will have to pay the remaining 30 percent. The Silver plan will cost slightly more than the Bronze plan. The Silver plan is a good choice for people who may have a few healthcare issues but are unlikely to use many services.

The **Gold plan** splits all covered expenses 80-20. The Gold plan monthly premium is going to cost more than the Silver plan; however, you and your family will likely be able to get the healthcare they need and will be able to afford the out-of-pocket costs.

The **Platinum plan** splits all covered expenses 90-10. This plan will have the highest per-month premium. This plan might be the best choice for someone who has a known illness and is likely to need significant healthcare services.

The last choice is a **Catastrophic plan**. This plan is only available to people under the age of 30 or who have a hardship exemption. A Catastrophic plan has very few benefits and a very limited network of hospitals and doctors. There will be high out-of-pocket costs and high deductibles. This plan merely protects you from the possibility that you might get very sick or be in an accident and need hospitalization. A Catastrophic plan does not include any of the required "basics" that must be in all the other ObamaCare health insurance plans.

### How Do I Pick a Plan that is Right for Me?

In choosing a plan, you must balance the monthly premium against the yearly deductible. Normally, if you choose a higher deductible your premium will be lower. If you believe that you are likely to need a lot of healthcare services, it is better to pick a higher premium with a lower deductible. Remember, preventative care, which includes regular checkups and screenings, is always exempt from the deductible.

Each plan is required to provide a **Summary of Benefits.** The Summary of Benefits will detail the specifics of the plan. It will list the overall deductible, your out-of-pocket limit, whether the plan requires you to receive services in a specific network, and whether you need a referral to see a specialist, among other things. Be certain to review the Summary of Benefits prior to purchasing the plan.

If it is important that you keep your current doctor, you should call his or her office to see if he or she is in the network of your potential new health insurance plan. If your doctor is either not within the network or does not accept this insurance plan, you might consider a different plan.

While some individuals will have a range of choices available to them, others will not. In some areas of the country, there are very limited choices for health plans. This may be because health insurance companies did not want to participate in your area or there may be very little competition in your healthcare market. Again, each state will vary as to what plans are offered.

### What Do I Do If I Picked the Wrong Plan?

In most circumstances, once you pick a plan you will not be able to switch that plan until the next **open enrollment period**. The only time you may be able to change plans is when you have not yet paid the first month's premium. So, it is very important to review all aspects of the plans before you choose one.

The first open enrollment period for the exchanges was very long, ending on March 31, 2014, due in part to the delay in getting the federal healthcare exchange to work properly. If you did not buy insurance by March 31, 2014, you will not be able to purchase until the next open enrollment, beginning November 15, 2014, and running through January 15, 2015. In the following years, the open enrollment period will be much shorter, running from October 15th through December 7th of each year.

## "LIFE-EVENTS" ALLOW YOU TO ENROLL OR DIS-ENROLL

Many events arise in life when your healthcare needs change. For example, you might have a baby so you need to add him or her to your plan in the middle of the year. These types of circumstances create a **"special enrollment period"** under ObamaCare. If you qualify, you will be permitted to buy health insurance or change your health plan during this special enrollment period. You must have had a specific change in your life in order to qualify. Getting sick will not qualify you for enrolling in health insurance outside of the open enrollment period.

For example, losing your existing employer-provided health insurance usually creates a special enrollment period. However, if you lose your existing health insurance because you did not pay the premiums, you will not be eligible for a special enrollment. Other changes such as getting married, divorced, having a baby, or adopting a child qualify for a special enrollment period. You might also have gotten a job that includes health benefits. Therefore, you would be entitled to dis-enroll from your ObamaCare plan during the special enrollment period.

Other circumstances such as permanently relocating can also create a special enrollment period. This also applies to people being released from prison. Special enrollment periods are only open for 30 days from the time of the "life event." For example, if you lost your job on July 1, you would have to enroll in an ObamaCare health insurance plan within 30 days from July 1st. Once 30 days have passed, you will have to wait until the next open enrollment to change your health plan or buy health insurance if you are uninsured.

If you do not have a "qualified" health insurance plan by the end of the enrollment period, you will be required to pay a penalty for remaining uninsured.

### WAITING PERIODS

It is important to understand that health insurance coverage does not take effect the day you buy it. Normally, if you sign up for insurance before the 15th of the month, your coverage will start at the beginning of the next month. If you enroll after the 15th of the month, your coverage will likely take effect the beginning of the month following the next month. For example, if you sign up on March 20th, your coverage will take effect May 1st.

### OBAMACARE PROVIDES PREMIUM CAPS BASED ON YOUR INCOME

ObamaCare provides a limit to how much you can be charged for your monthly health insurance premium based on your income. For example, if your income is between 300 percent and 400 percent of the federal poverty level, you can only be charged up to 9.5 percent of your income for your health insurance premium. The premium caps are only based on the Silver Plan cost so if you choose a higher-level plan you have to make up the difference.

### Navigators

Going to an on-line healthcare exchange or marketplace is not the only way to sign up for insurance coverage. ObamaCare provides for health insurance **"navigators"** to inform people about their rights under ObamaCare and to assist them in signing up for a plan that works best for them. A navigator will also help resolve any problems you might have with your enrollment or health insurance coverage. Navigators do not receive any commission from health insurance companies. Therefore, they tend to provide objective advice. This is different from insurance brokers who will receive a commission from the plan their customers choose. If you are looking for a navigator in your state, you should contact your state's health department to get a list of navigators. The federal government gave out a number of grants to a variety of non-profit groups to hire and train navigators, so most navigators work for those organizations.

It is important to remember that there are many ways to enroll in ObamaCare. Enrollment can be done on the phone, in person through a navigator, or on-line.

# THE BOTTOM LINE...

- Some states will have a state health exchange and others will not.

- If your state does not have a health exchange, you will use the federal health exchange.

- All insurance plans on the exchanges will cover certain basic services.

- There are five types of plans to choose from: Bronze, Silver, Gold, Platinum, and Catastrophic.

- Each plan will have different co-pays and deductibles depending on what you choose.

- Once you pay for the premium, you will not be able to choose a different plan until the next enrollment period.

- Life events (getting married, losing your job, having a baby, etc.) may allow you to sign up or change your insurance outside of the open enrollment period.

- A waiting period will normally occur prior to your insurance taking effect.

- You may be eligible for a premium cap based on your income.

- Navigators can assist you in selecting the plan that is right for you.

# 7.

# WHO IS ELIGIBLE FOR A TAX SUBSIDY?

Starting in 2014, tax subsidies came into play to assist some in paying for their healthcare coverage. Tax subsidies are available to individuals and families who cannot otherwise get health insurance coverage. This includes those who are within 100 percent to 400 percent of the poverty line. In 2014, 400 percent of the poverty line equaled $47,000 for an individual and $96,000 for a family of four.

Unlike most tax credits, the ObamaCare tax subsidy is paid directly to the health insurance company in real time (in other words, you do not wait until you file your federal tax return to take the credit). Therefore, many individuals will not have to pay their insurance premiums each month since the tax subsidy may cover the cost. Also, depending on your ability to pay, you will be eligible for decreased co-pays and deductibles.

It is important to remember that tax subsidies are based on a projection of your income for the year. If, for some reason, your income changes and you make more than what you originally projected, you will be required to pay back the federal government for the portion of the tax subsidies you should not have received.

## MEDICAID ELIGIBILITY AND THE TAX SUBSIDY

You will only be entitled to tax subsidies if your income is above the federal poverty line. This is because the lawmakers who passed ObamaCare envisioned that all individuals living below the poverty line would be eligible for Medicaid as part of an expansion of the program under the new law. Therefore these individuals would not have to buy insurance on the exchanges. In 2012, however, the U.S. Supreme Court made Medicaid expansion optional for states. So, if you live in a state that has chosen not to expand Medicaid and you are below the federal poverty line, you can buy insurance on the health exchange; however, you will not be eligible for tax subsidies.

## *How Do I Apply for a Tax Subsidy and How Much Will It Be?*

You apply for a tax subsidy directly from the health insurance exchange. If you purchase your insurance from somewhere other than a health exchange, you will want to make sure that you are buying a qualified plan that will allow you to obtain the appropriate tax subsidies.

In order to determine how much your tax subsidy will be, you will need to know two things. First, you will need to know your expected contribution toward the cost of your healthcare. Second, you will need to know the cost of your benchmark health plan. Your health insurance exchange can tell you which plan this is and how much it costs. Your benchmark plan is the Silver health plan with the second lowest monthly premium in your area. Your subsidy amount is the difference between your expected contribution and the cost of your benchmark health plan. You do not need to purchase the benchmark health plan if it does not meet your needs. The benchmark health plan is merely used to calculate your tax subsidy. If you purchase a more expensive health plan, your tax subsidy remains the same.

# THE BOTTOM LINE...

- Depending on your income, you may receive tax subsidies that will pay all or a portion of your monthly health insurance premium.

- Your tax subsidy will be paid directly to the insurance company each month.

- Some low-income individuals will not be eligible for tax subsidies in states that have not expanded Medicaid.

- You can apply for your tax subsidy on your health exchange.

- Your tax subsidy will be the difference between your expected contribution and the cost of your benchmark health plan.

# 8.

# WHAT IS MEDICAID EXPANSION?

When ObamaCare was first passed, it required states to expand their Medicaid program to include more individuals. However, in 2012, the U.S. Supreme Court determined that states were not required to expand their Medicaid programs. So, some states have chosen to expand Medicaid and others have not.

As envisioned by the lawmakers who created Obamacare, Medicaid expansion was intended to address two issues: increase medical coverage of the working poor and decrease the use of emergency healthcare services. Many uninsured individuals do not address medical conditions until they become emergencies since they cannot afford regular doctor's visits, preventative care, or ongoing treatments. Emergency room visits and the resulting hospital stays are very expensive and often go unpaid by the uninsured patient. Unpaid bills to hospitals are one of the main causes for the increased cost of healthcare.

## What is Medicaid?

Medicaid is a joint federal- and state-funded program that provides healthcare to over 60 million low-income Americans. The program defines low income as being within a certain yearly income range compared to the federal poverty line. Before ObamaCare, Medicaid primarily covered impoverished children, their parents, and pregnant women as well as people with disabilities and the elderly who needed assistance or lived in nursing homes. But Medicaid did not cover adults who were without dependent children or disabilities. Therefore, most low-income adults under 65 were not entitled to Medicaid prior to Medicaid expansion under ObamaCare.

People with Medicaid do not pay a monthly premium for their health insurance due to their low-income levels. This is different from an individual with a higher income who does not have health insurance. The higher income individual will purchase their insurance from the health exchange and will be required to pay a monthly premium.

## IF MY STATE EXPANDS MEDICAID, WHO WILL BE COVERED?

Medicaid expansion increases Medicaid eligibility to all individuals and families below 100 percent to 138 percent of the federal poverty line. Now, for the first time, low-income adults with or without dependent children will be eligible for Medicaid coverage. Low-income children who lose their Medicaid benefits when they become adults will remain eligible for Medicaid. Further, low-income adults with disabilities who are not eligible for Social Security will be eligible for Medicaid. Thus, Medicaid expansion will cover many individuals who were not previously covered by the program. While specific eligibility details are determined on a state-by-state basis, the federal government dictates certain minimum requirements.

Starting in 2014, states that have expanded Medicaid must increase eligibility levels to $11,670 for an individual and $23,850 for a family of four. Depending on your state, individuals with incomes up to $15,521 and families up to $31,721 may be eligible for Medicaid. Prior to ObamaCare, every state had different Medicaid eligibility requirements based on income, age, gender, dependence, and other specific state requirements. If your state is now expanding Medicaid, it will have the same eligibility requirements as all the other states that are expanding Medicaid.

Most individuals covered by Medicaid before ObamaCare had no income at all. Medicaid expansion, however, will cover those families who are considered the working poor. Often, poor working families cannot afford health insurance because it is too expensive. Medicaid expansion is meant to cover the gap between those people who do not meet current Medicaid eligibility and those who can afford subsidized private insurance through the health exchange. It is estimated that about half of the uninsured in America would be covered by Medicaid expansion if all states chose to participate.

## IF MY STATE EXPANDS MEDICAID, WHO WILL PAY FOR IT?

Any state that chooses to expand Medicaid will receive 100 percent funding from the federal government in 2016 and 90 percent coverage for the cost of expansion in subsequent years. For those states that have not expanded Medicaid, the federal government will not increase the federal portion of the state's Medicaid funding.

## DID MY STATE EXPAND MEDICAID?

As of 2014, twenty-five states and the District of Columbia have chosen to expand Medicaid. The states that have chosen expansion are: Arizona, Arkansas, California, Colorado, Connecticut, Delaware, Hawaii, Illinois, Iowa, Kentucky, Maryland, Massachusetts, Michigan, Minnesota, Nevada, New Jersey, New Mexico, New York, North Dakota, Ohio, Oregon, Rhode Island, Vermont, Washington, and West Virginia.

The states that have chosen not to expand Medicare as of 2014 are: Alabama, Alaska, Georgia, Florida, Idaho, Indiana, Kansas, Louisiana, Maine, Mississippi, Montana, Nebraska, North Carolina, Oklahoma, South Carolina, South Dakota, Tennessee, Texas, Virginia, Wyoming, and Wisconsin. The states that have not expanded Medicaid but are considering doing so are: Missouri, New Hampshire, Pennsylvania, and Utah.

There is a vast difference in services depending on what state you live in. If you live in a state that has expanded Medicaid, you are likely to have Medicaid coverage if you earn up to $31,809 for a family of four. If you live in a state that is not expanding Medicaid, you may have the same income but not have coverage.

### WHAT IF MY STATE DID NOT EXPAND MEDICAID?

If your state did not expand Medicaid, the program that existed prior to ObamaCare is still in place. However, many individuals who would have been covered in an expansion, such as some low-income parents, will not be. For example, if your state only allows parents with dependent children to be eligible for Medicaid if their median income is 48 percent of the federal poverty line, they will not be eligible for Medicaid if their income is more than that amount. Likewise, they will not be eligible for tax subsidies on a healthcare exchange until their median income is above the federal poverty line.

### CAN I BUY INSURANCE FROM THE HEALTH EXCHANGE IF MY STATE HASN'T EXPANDED MEDICAID?

If you live in a state without Medicaid expansion, you may still be eligible to purchase insurance through a health exchange if your income is more than 100 percent of the poverty line. In 2014, the poverty line is $11,670 per year for one person or $23,850 for a family of four.

### MEDICAID PAYMENTS AND SERVICES EXPANDED

ObamaCare also addressed some of the complaints made about Medicaid in the past. For example, many doctors will not accept Medicaid due to its low payment rates. ObamaCare does increase Medicaid payments to the same level as Medicare payments. Also preventative services are now covered under ObamaCare. These services include tests for high blood pressure, diabetes, and high cholesterol. Many cancer screenings, including colonoscopies and mammograms, are also now covered. Medicaid will also now cover counseling to assist people in losing weight, quitting smoking, and reducing alcohol use. Routine vaccinations are also covered.

# THE BOTTOM LINE...

- ObamaCare expanded Medicaid to include more low-income individuals.

- The U.S. Supreme Court determined that states could decide whether they want to expand Medicaid or not.

- If a state expands Medicaid, it will cover low-income individuals without dependents.

- If your state expands Medicaid, the federal government will mostly pay for the costs of the expansion.

- If you live in a state that did not expand Medicaid, you may have the same income as individuals living in Medicaid expansion states but not have coverage.

- Under ObamaCare, Medicaid services have been expanded to include preventative services, higher payments to doctors, and preventative screenings.

# 9.

# HOW DOES OBAMACARE AFFECT EMPLOYEES COVERED BY EMPLOYER-SPONSORED HEALTH INSURANCE

As we discussed above, if you have an employer-provided health plan, you will not be eligible for healthcare plans on the exchanges. However, ObamaCare does include some rules that may affect employees with employer-provided healthcare. For employers with more than 50 employees, ObamaCare requires that the employer provide insurance to the employees or pay a penalty starting in 2015. Also, insurance must be provided to any employee who works more than 30 hours. Therefore some employers have limited employees' hours to less than 30 hours in order to avoid providing health insurance.

Also, starting in 2016, your employer's health plan must, in most circumstances, meet the basic essential elements defined under ObamaCare. There are some exceptions, which were discussed above. In 2015, your employer must also show on your paycheck how much the company pays for your health coverage.

## "Cadillac" Health Plans

Another part of the ObamaCare law taxes an employer who provides an expensive "Cadillac" health plan to its employees. In 2018, the rule will impose a 40 percent excise tax on employee benefits that exceed $10,200 for individuals and $27,500 for families. In 2013, the average employer-sponsored health plan for individuals cost $5,884 and the average family plan cost $16,351. Therefore the Cadillac tax will only impact a small number of employers.

## Small Business Benefits

Small employers who were not able to provide health insurance on their own may shop on the health exchange to locate affordable coverage for their employees. The **Small Business Health Options Program (SHOP)** provides small businesses with the opportunity to pool their risks together in order to have access to more insurers, greater options, and lower costs. Prior to the implementation of ObamaCare, small businesses paid 18 percent more for health insurance than larger businesses. In order to be eligible to participate in SHOP, a small business must:

- offer coverage to all its full-time employees

- have 70 percent of those full-time employees actually enroll in the plan

- participate in a SHOP that is within the geographical service area of its office or workplace

The small business might also be eligible for healthcare tax credits. A small business with fewer than 25 full-time employees can receive a tax credit of up to 50 percent of the amount it pays toward insuring its employees. The small business will be eligible to receive a tax credit if it (1) pays at least 50 percent of the cost of single healthcare coverage for a full-time employee; (2) their employees earn, on average, less than $50,000 a year; and (3) the insurance plan is bought through a SHOP.

The small business can also implement workplace wellness programs based on the guidelines outlined in ObamaCare. Wellness programs incentivize healthy behavior by employees through rewards given to the employee for meeting health-related goals. For example the employer can reward an employee for losing weight, lowering cholesterol, or stopping smoking. The maximum reward is 30 percent of the cost of health coverage or 50 percent if the goal relates to smoking.

# *THE BOTTOM LINE...*

- Employees who receive healthcare insurance from their employer will not be eligible to buy insurance on the exchanges.

- Employers with more than 50 employees must offer health insurance to all full-time employees.

- Employers who provide expensive health plans may have to pay a tax on those plans.

- Small businesses that previously could not offer health insurance to employees may now be able to purchase insurance on the exchanges.

- ObamaCare rules support workplace wellness programs.

- Small businesses may be entitled to tax credits if they provide employee health insurance.

# 10.

# WHAT'S THE PENALTY FOR NOT BUYING HEALTH INSURANCE?

For those individuals who choose not to buy insurance, they will be subject to a penalty.

### HOW MUCH IS THE PENALTY?

Patients who can afford health insurance are required to buy insurance or pay a $95 penalty or one percent of their income, whichever is greater in 2014. Currently, the cost of unpaid medical care for people who choose to remain uninsured is passed on to everyone paying for health insurance. Thus, ObamaCare requires each person who remains uninsured to pay some of the costs of the uncompensated care.

If you choose to remain uninsured, you might prefer to pay the healthcare penalty, as it will likely be cheaper than the insurance premium you might have to pay in 2014. For example, the average monthly price for a Silver plan will generally be $200-$300 a month. Thus, the penalty may be cheaper than the premium in 2014. This is especially true for those people who are not entitled to a tax subsidy to assist in paying for the monthly premium.

For example, a person making $50,000 a year would not be eligible for a subsidy and would have to pay the full price for the premium, typically $2,400-$3,600 a year. If the individual making $50,000 a year declined health insurance, he would only be subject to a $400 penalty for 2014. This of course assumes that the individual will have no healthcare costs that would otherwise be paid for by health insurance.

Compare the above individual example to a couple jointly earning $50,000 a year. The couple would receive a $1,300 subsidy, leaving them to pay about $4,750 in premiums for the year. The same couple would pay a $300 penalty if they chose not to buy insurance. So, if you feel you will not have a lot of medical expenses, it may be preferable to pay the penalty.

Also, the penalty is prorated if people purchase insurance coverage for part of the year. There will be no penalty if you lack coverage for less than a three-month period during the year.

## PENALTIES WILL INCREASE

The amount of the penalty increases over time. For 2014, the flat fee is $95 per adult and $47.50 per child, up to $285 per family or one percent of the family income, whichever is larger. Income is defined as total income above the filing threshold, which is $10,000 for an individual and $20,000 for a family in 2014. So, a person making $50,000 would be subject to a $400 penalty, while a couple earning that amount would each pay $300.

By 2016, the flat fee grows quickly to $695 per adult and $347.50 per child or 2.5 percent of family income, whichever is larger. However, the penalty is limited so that it cannot exceed the national average premium for a Bronze Plan in the state-based exchanges. Thus, by 2016, it may be cheaper to buy insurance then to pay the penalty. This limit encourages people to buy insurance rather than spend their money paying a penalty.

## SOME PEOPLE ARE EXEMPT FROM THE PENALTY

Certain individuals are exempt from the penalty. If you do not pay any federal taxes, you will not have to pay a penalty for failing to buy health insurance. Additionally, undocumented immigrants and Native Americans are exempt from the penalty. Also exempt are people who pay more than eight percent of their income for health insurance and poor adults who live in states that are not expanding Medicaid. The uninsured can also file for a hardship exemption to avoid the penalty.

## HOW ARE PENALTIES COLLECTED?

The penalties are collected through your tax return. It will be difficult, however, for the Internal Revenue Service (IRS) to collect the penalty. As of 2014, the IRS has no authority to prosecute anyone who fails to pay the penalty. However, the IRS can withhold the penalty from any refund that is due.

## *THE BOTTOM LINE...*

- In 2014, an individual will have to pay a $95 penalty or one percent or their income, whichever is greater, if they do not have insurance.

- Penalties will increase each year through 2016.

- The penalty cannot exceed the average premium for a Bronze plan.

- Some people will be exempt from the penalty.

- Penalties will be collected through your tax return.

# Conclusion

ObamaCare is a "starting point" to address some very basic problems in healthcare. It certainly isn't perfect and will require many significant adjustments over time. Whether you are for or against it, everyone should understand the basics of the law and how it affects them and their loved ones. Indeed, ObamaCare will continue to make significant changes to healthcare and the health insurance industry for years to come. As the healthcare industry responds to these changes, consumers will need to be vigilant in order to receive the care they need and deserve. And HealthSpin will be there to help make sense of it.

# TERMS TO KNOW

**Accountable Care Organization (ACO):** Instituted by the Affordable Care Act, a group of physicians who join together to improve quality and better coordinate care under Medicare.

**Affordable Care Act:** See Patient Protection and Affordable Care Act (ACA).

**Bronze plan:** Health insurance plan on the health insurance exchange that pays 60 percent of an individual's healthcare costs. Bronze plans have the most basic benefits and will likely have the most limited network of doctors and hospitals.

**Catastrophic plan:** Health insurance plan on the health insurance exchange that is only available to individuals under the age of 30 or who have a hardship exemption. Catastrophic plans have very few benefits and a very limited network of hospitals and doctors and are intended to protect individuals in the event of a sudden serious illness, hospitalization, or accident.

**Clinical trial:** Research study that uses human participants to answer specific health questions. Examples include drug trials and studies measuring the effect of certain behaviors on overall health.

**Coinsurance:** Similar to a co-pay, a percentage of the cost of the actual procedure as opposed to a flat fee.

**Community Care Transitions Plan (CCTP):** Program implemented in 2011 under ObamaCare and running for five years designed to keep high-risk Medicare patients from returning to the hospital by connecting them with services in their communities such as a home health agency.

**Co-pay:** Flat fee an individual pays as an "out of pocket" expense when he or she visits the doctor.

**Deductible:** The amount an individual must spend before a health insurance plan will make payments for his or her healthcare. Some services, for example preventative care, are exempt from the deductible.

**Donut hole:** Term referring to the gap in Medicare Part D coverage that occurs when seniors exceed their yearly limit on prescription drug costs.

**Electronic Health Record (EHR):** A digital record that includes your name, address, age, social security number, medical history, immunizations, allergies, medications, laboratory results, radiology imaging, personal information, and billing information. May also be called an "electronic medical record."

**Fee for service:** Financial model in which physicians charge and are paid a "fee" for each service they provide regardless of patient outcomes. A fee may be charged for an office visit, a procedure, a test, etc.

**Flat rate payment:** Financial model in which a hospital, group of healthcare providers, and post-acute care facilities are paid one flat fee for an "episode" of care for a patient.

**Gold plan:** Health insurance plan on the health insurance exchange that pays 80 percent of an individual's healthcare costs. Gold plans are intended for those who have several healthcare issues and are likely to use several services.

**Health insurance exchange:** Mandated by the Affordable Care Act, an online site where individuals can shop for and buy healthcare insurance. The federal health insurance exchange is www.healthcare.gov.

**Independent Payment Advisory Board (IPAB):** Fifteen-member panel created by the Affordable Care Act made up of non-practicing physicians, healthcare policy experts, healthcare facilities managers, health service researchers, employers, consumers and representatives for the elderly. This board has limited authority to make proposals designed to curb the overall cost of Medicare if it becomes uncontrollable. However, the IPAB is specifically barred from recommending cuts to healthcare that threaten Medicare beneficiaries' access to care. Not formed as of 2014.

**In Network:** Term used to describe doctors and hospitals that accept the contracted rate of an insurance plan, which is often less than what they would normally charge.

**Lifetime limit:** Maximum dollar amount an insurance company would pay on an individual. Once this limit was reached, the insurance company would end coverage. Under ObamaCare, lifetime limits are no longer allowed.

**Medicaid:** A joint federal- and state-funded program that provides healthcare to low-income Americans.

**Medicaid Expansion:** A provision in the Affordable Care Act mandating that states expand their existing Medicaid programs to cover a larger number of individuals living at or below the federal poverty line. However, in 2012, the U.S. Supreme Court ruled that Medicare expansion was not mandatory for states. Therefore Medicaid expansion has only occurred in a limited number of states.

**Medicare:** Insurance program run by the federal government that provides health coverage to people over the age of 65. Medicare also provides coverage for people with certain disabilities as well as those with end stage renal disease.

**Medicare Advantage:** Health insurance offered to seniors by private companies and approved by Medicare.

**Navigator:** Mandated by the Affordable Care Act, individuals who assist others in understanding their rights under the law, in selecting a health insurance plan, and addressing any problems that might arise during enrollment. Navigators generally work for non-profits and do not receive any commissions.

**ObamaCare:** See Patient Protection and Affordable Care Act (ACA).

**Open Enrollment Period:** Span of time in which an individual can purchase a healthcare plan on the health insurance exchanges.

**Out of network:** Term used to describe doctors and hospitals that do not accept the contracted rate of an insurance plan.

**Out-of-pocket costs:** Costs associated with health insurance plans that are paid by the individual themselves and not the insurance provider.

**Out-of-pocket maximum:** The highest amount an individual will have to pay for healthcare in a year as part of a health insurance plan.

**Patient Protection and Affordable Care Act (ACA):** Federal law signed by President Barack Obama in 2010 that fundamentally reformed the U.S. healthcare system and the health insurance industry.

**Platinum plan:** Health insurance plan on the health insurance exchange that pays 90 percent of an individual's healthcare costs. Platinum plans are intended for those who have serious healthcare issues and will be significant consumers of healthcare services.

**Pre-existing condition:** A health issue that existed (or currently exists) before you apply for insurance coverage. A pre-existing condition may include a chronic condition such as diabetes or a previous illness such as cancer.

**Premium:** The monthly price an individual pays to have access to his or her health insurance plan.

**Preventative care:** Medical procedures and practices, such as annual physicals and health screenings such as colonoscopies and mammograms, that aid in keeping a patient healthy by identifying serious illnesses early and promoting good habits.

**Recovery and Reinvestment Act:** Legislation signed into law by President Barak Obama that used tax cuts, increased federal spending, and social welfare funding to stimulate the economy.

**Silver plan:** Health insurance plan on the health insurance exchange that pays 70 percent of an individual's healthcare costs. Silver plans are intended for those who have a few healthcare issues but are unlikely to use many services.

**Small Business Health Options Program (SHOP):** Program created by the Affordable Care Act that provides small businesses the opportunity to pool their risks together in order to have access to more insurers, greater options and lower costs when purchasing a healthcare plan for their employees.

**Special Enrollment Period:** Span of time outside of the normal enrollment period when an individual can purchase or change his or her health insurance plan due to a major life change, such as marriage, divorce, job loss, or having a baby.

**Summary of Benefits.** Document that outlines the specifics of a healthcare plan, including the overall deductible, out-of-pocket limit, whether the plan requires you to receive services in a specific network, and whether you need a referral to see a specialist, etc.

# LORI-ANN'S ON YOUR SIDE

"When I need health care advice I can understand and
follow, I call Lori-Ann. She knows her stuff!"
*M. Diane Vogt, JD*

"Lori-Ann is my "go-to" expert on healthcare law.
She makes it understandable and easy to follow
for our doctors and their patients, too."
*Michele Nichols, The Physician Alliance*

"Lori-Ann knows the healthcare system inside and out.  Whenever
we have questions about healthcare, Lori-Ann has the answers."
*Mike Gerstenlauer, St. John-Macomb Hospital*

"Whenever my family has a health care issue, Lori-
Ann is my first call for the best advice."
*Donna Curran*

"Getting coverage for prescription drugs can be a big problem for
patients. Lori-Ann knows the insider secrets to making it easy."
*Coreen Buehrer*

"Lori-Ann has also lived the difficult issues that families confront on
a daily basis as they struggle with the bewildering maze of hospitals,
multiple specialists and insurance companies as our family's tire-
less advocate for our father.  No mother grizzly ever fought for her
cubs with more passion than Lori-Ann looked out for our dad."
*Stephen Rickard, J.D., MPA*

# ABOUT THE AUTHOR

Lori-Ann Rickard is one of the country's top healthcare lawyers. For over three decades, she has advised leading hospitals, doctors, laboratories, and other healthcare providers. Now she offers her expertise to patients and their families through the Easy Healthcare Series from HealthSpin.

Lori-Ann is also a single mom of two beautiful daughters. One of her daughters was very sick when she was born. Already caring for a toddler and managing a developing career, Lori-Ann used her professional experience to create quick, effective strategies to make the healthcare system work for her as she sought the best treatment possible for her sick baby. Later, Lori-Ann served as the primary caregiver and medical coordinator for her proud, independent parents when they became unable to care for themselves. Through their wellness challenges, her daughter's illness, and in helping friends over the past thirty years, Lori-Ann has used her unique position in the industry to create easy healthcare solutions that work for everyone around her. These solutions will work for you and your family, too.

Lori-Ann Rickard is a healthcare insider who knows what it means to be a patient and a caregiver. The Easy Healthcare Series brings you the benefit of Lori-Ann Rickard's expertise. Let her show you how you can Spin Your Healthcare Your Way.

# MORE BY LORI-ANN RICKARD

Visit myhealthspin.com to download your free copy
of *Easy Healthcare: What You Need First!*
ALSO AVAILABLE FROM HEALTHSPIN:

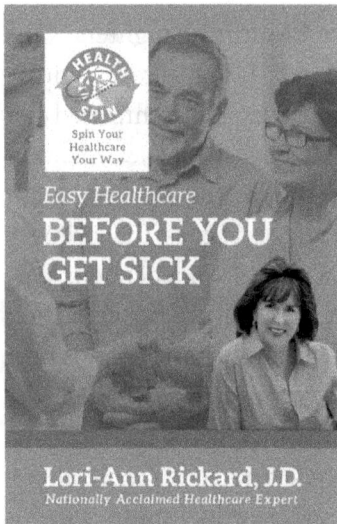

HEALTH SPIN

Spin Your
Healthcare
Your Way

*Easy Healthcare*

**BEFORE YOU
GET SICK**

Lori-Ann Rickard, J.D.
Nationally Acclaimed Healthcare Expert

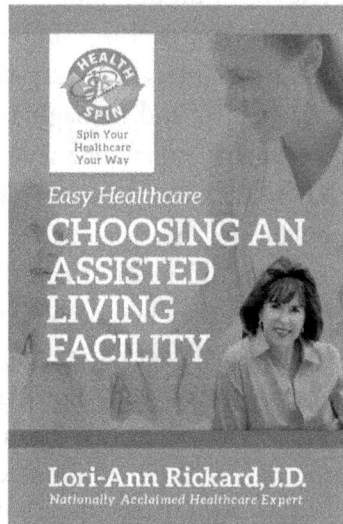

HEALTH SPIN

Spin Your
Healthcare
Your Way

*Easy Healthcare*

**CHOOSING AN
ASSISTED
LIVING
FACILITY**

Lori-Ann Rickard, J.D.
Nationally Acclaimed Healthcare Expert

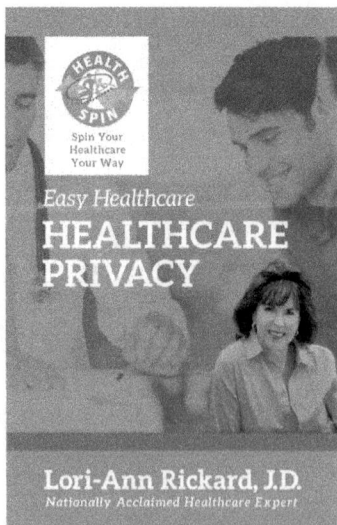

HEALTH SPIN

Spin Your
Healthcare
Your Way

*Easy Healthcare*

**HEALTHCARE
PRIVACY**

Lori-Ann Rickard, J.D.
Nationally Acclaimed Healthcare Expert

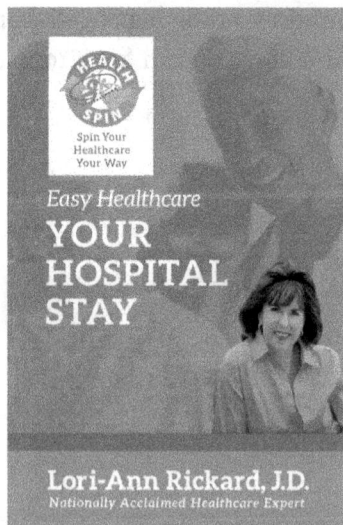

HEALTH SPIN

Spin Your
Healthcare
Your Way

*Easy Healthcare*

**YOUR
HOSPITAL
STAY**

Lori-Ann Rickard, J.D.
Nationally Acclaimed Healthcare Expert

www.ingramcontent.com/pod-product-compliance
Lightning Source LLC
Chambersburg PA
CBHW050602280326
41933CB00011B/1948